<u>CONTENTS</u>

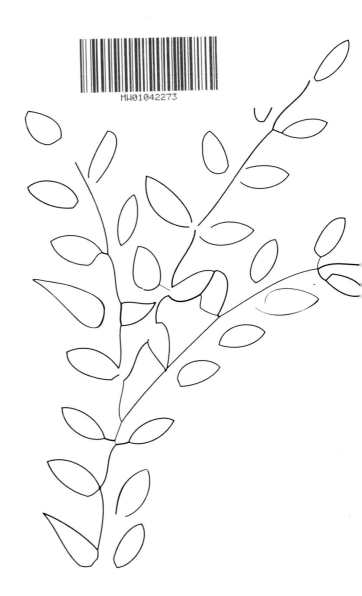

"Thou anointest my head with oil; my cup runneth over."

-King James Version, Psalm 23:5

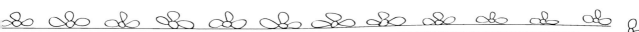

Welcome to *"The Art of Centering"* using Wall Yoga

Wall Yoga allows you to use the stability of the ground, the wall, and accessories, to center and maintain a solid and powerful asana. Proper alignment involves being able to root and ground the foundation of your asana. When you do, you are able to experience lightness, openness and flexibility in each yoga pose.

As an instructor, I find my students make the most progress in learning a new asana when they are able to approach it with strength and confidence. First, find a place that offers wall and floor space.

It would be nice to have available the following items:
- A Yoga Mat
- Yoga Soft Blocks
- Yoga Knots
- Therapy Ball
- Yoga Gloves

I encourage the use of accessories. These wonderful tools help students achieve their goals quickly. Early success leads to more enjoyment and greater control as you approach each asana. There is a reference guide where you will find my favorite accessories and recommended vendors at the end of this book. These items are also available at www.wallyogaworkout.com. I have included several pages, to show you a complete yoga flow, day–by–day progress charts, and how to perform the classic Sun Salutation.

When you begin your yoga session, step onto the mat with a healthy and grateful attitude. Be grateful you are physically able to set time aside to care for your body and mind. Acknowledge the amazing power of becoming centered and balanced. Keep this favorable attitude throughout your yoga session.

Remember, in yoga, the body works as a whole. The beauty of applying the Wall in yoga is to allow you to maintain a steadier and more accurate asana. When you are secure in your asana, your mind has more time to imprint the image and develop correct muscle memory.

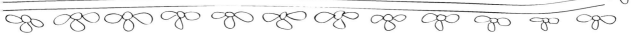

Note to Deaf and Hard of Hearing Students

I was born into a family of five out of seven children with nerve deafness. I wanted those who desire to make yoga part of their life to be able to do so, whether hearing or deaf.

At www.wallyogaworkout.com, you can request interpreting services for deaf or hard of hearing students. Yoga changes lives. Everyone, hearing or deaf, deserves to incorporate this powerful healing antidote into their lives, no matter what obstacles they face.

Feel free to drop me a line. I would love to hear from you!

Namaste,

Colette Barry, L.M.T.
Certified Yoga, Pilates, & Thai Yoga Instructor

www.wallyogaworkout.com
Colette@wallyogaworkout.com

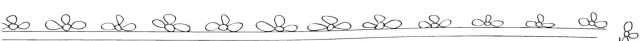

 Getting the most out of your "Wall Yoga" book

In this section, we'll clarify specific guidelines and descriptions used throughout the book. Yoga is to be embraced first with your heart.

Be prepared and open to changes physically, mentally and spiritually. Anticipate an adventure of a lifetime. When you put Yoga in your life, your life will become a very satifying experience.

The Five—Week Program

The "Art of Centering" is a five-week program. Follow the Wall Yoga program by observing the pattern of the borders on the workout series pages.

Week 1   Week 2   Week 3   Week 4   Week 5

Each week consists of four pages. Each page teaches a specific asana. Within each page there is an "Advanced" asana, which is optional for those who desire more of a challenge.

By following the series week by week, you will work every muscle group in your body. In 30 days you will build a solid core, develop a mobile spine, release tension between the joints and begin to obtain long lean muscles.

Once you have finished all 5 weeks, return to week 1 and repeat the cycle. Stay with the program and aches and pains will begin to disappear. **You'll have more energy, and feel more tranquility in your daily life.** Visit us online and become a member at ww.wallyogaworkout.com. There, you can watch each asana from this book demonstrated on video. I explain body positioning and how to achieve maximum benefits from the workout.

Symbols and Images

Drishti

Drishti derives from the word *dris* in Sanskrit meaning "to see" also known as "gazing point." When engaging into an asana, Drishti help to quiet your mind and pull you into focus.

Throughout Wall Yoga, each asana includes a small symbol under each description. These images offer suggestions on where to focus your gaze. Remember to gaze softly and without straining. It's important to keep your mind quiet and focused while practicing your asana. Wandering eyes can cause an unfocused mind.

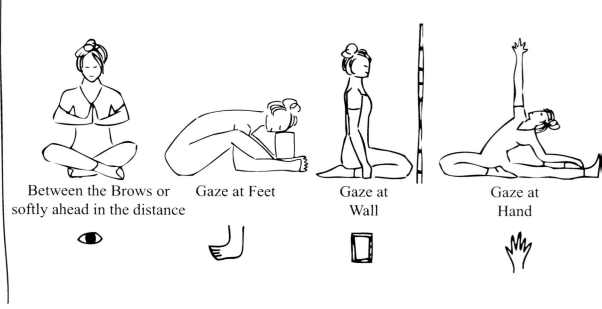

Between the Brows or softly ahead in the distance

Gaze at Feet

Gaze at Wall

Gaze at Hand

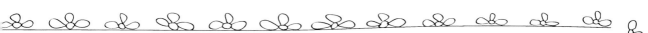

 Grounding Your Poses with Accessories

Throughout Wall Yoga, I offer various poses that involve stabilizing your asana with Yoga Knots, Blocks, Therapy Balls, and of course, the Wall. When used they create a stable and balanced pose. When we physically touch an object to root our asana, we are establishing a number of things:

- Beginners and advanced students benefit from using accessories since they help obtain a better asana. A more aligned asana means more powerful results.

- Using accessories creates a sense of security and stability in a pose. When your body feels secure and stable, your muscles begin to relax. As your muscles relax, you develop flexibility. When accessories are applied, your mind can turn its focus on surrendering where tension and strain begin to disappear.

- Accessories help you prevent fatiguing prematurely. When your body and mind can repeat the correct posture, you don't develop bad habits.

- Using yoga knots can help you grip your pose and loosen tight ligaments in shoulders and hips. Yoga Knots by Colette are designed in place of yoga straps to help you obtain a better grip in challenging poses. Various binding asana are extremely effective in allowing your body and mind to become grounded and centered.

- Finally, as this book implies, support is good. Using accessories in your yoga practice, gives you the ability to stretch deeper, bend farther, and align more accurately with less discomfort.

Once the muscles are trained and strengthened, the need for accessories diminishes.

Three Types of Accessories used in Wall Yoga

1. Therapy Ball

Ball work is an excellent exercise to help develop core muscles fast. In my Wall Yoga class, we practice with the ball because it creates another variation to strengthen and balance your muscles. To get results quickly, variation is the key. All the ball work poses in Wall Yoga are specifically chosen to give you a total body workout. You can find ball work in the following asana- Boat on Ball, Forward Bend with Wall and Ball, Lotus Pose with Ball, Lateral Incline Pose on Ball, and Plank on Ball.

Proper size of the ball is critical in getting the most out of your session. When you are seated on top of the ball your knees should be bent with your thighs parallel to the floor.

Your Height	Ball Size
5'1" to 5'6"	22 in
5'7" to 6'1"	26 in
6'2" to 6'8"	30 in
6'9" +	34 in

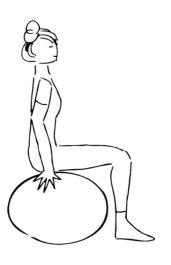

2. Yoga Blocks

To engage in your asana, you need to feel supported. To assure good support, Yoga Blocks are a must. Once your body becomes familiar with the poses and your muscles begin to strengthen, blocks will be unnecessary. Until then, use blocks to help establish proper body alignment from the beginning.

In my studio, we use Yoga Blocks that are soft yet supportive. Hard Yoga Blocks are painful when you use them to set or rest your head, which we do often in Wall Yoga. We use the Yoga Block size 3" x 6" x 9" most often. This is a nice size. It is easy to reach, yet not too large that it interferes with progression.

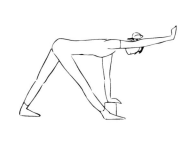

3. Yoga Knots

Yoga Knots were developed in my studio to help students obtain a stronger "grip" than the traditional yoga belt. A better grip helps "lock in" a tighter asana. This helps to stretch and lengthen the ligaments and muscle involved.

Knots or Belts are a terrific tool in helping you achieve greater mobility and "openness" in your shoulders and shoulder blades. They are instrumental when first learning to apply binding poses.

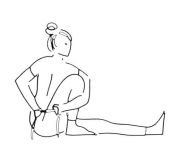

The Significance of Proper Alignment

Proper yoga alignment gives you the best results. That's why I designed this book. Using applications such as the Wall, Therapy Balls, Yoga Blocks and Yoga Knots helps you gain accuracy in your pose consistently. Accurate alignment allows your body to reap all the benefit yoga has to offer.

Breathing and proper alignment go hand and hand. When you pursue proper alignment, your chest fills **to capacity.** This provides fresh oxygen to all the cells in the body. Proper alignment helps maintain strong bones. It works every joint in your body. Strong muscles build strong joints. The body is restored to its natural state allowing mobility. Fluid movement means better flexibility throughout your entire body.

Like braces that help align your teeth, practicing accurate alignment through Wall Yoga rebuilds a healthy body and spine. Poor alignment is the source of many health complications. A misaligned body causes muscles to either over-compensate or under-compensate, putting excess stress on joints and ligaments. Eventually, healthy tissues begin to breakdown and joints become stiff and fragile.

The diagrams on the next pages illustrate two asana in proper and improper alignment. "The flat back" and "the mountain pose" are powerful examples of training your body to become properly aligned. They are the foundations of all other poses in this book. Practice these poses daily; use them as a guideline for all your other asana. Over time, your alignment will improve.

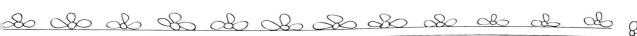

Proper Alignment

A- Proper Alignment of Flat Back
- Begin by using soft yoga blocks to practice building strong back muscles.
- Place feet perpendicular to the hips and hands perpendicular to the shoulders.
- With hands on soft blocks, focus eyes at a 45 degree angle from the floor. As the chin is raised, pull shoulders away from ears.
- Draw armpits down toward sides of hips.
- Press feet into floor then raise tailbone to ceiling.
- Last, pull shoulder blades down toward your lower back. Draw shoulder blades inward and downward.
- Hold this pose for 5 long steady breaths, allowing your mind to mirror this image and retain muscle memory. As the back muscles become stronger by applying this pose, your spine will realign and your body will become stronger and healthier.

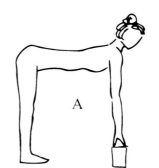

B- Improper Alignment of Flat Back
- Shoulders and shoulder blades are not drawn down toward hips, causing weakness of lateral and posterior muscles of the torso.
- Shoulders are close to ears caused by tight neck muscles.
- Upper back arching– caused by a weakened thoracic spine.
- The low back is arched posterior and the tailbone is pulled downward instead of upward.

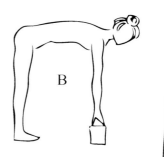

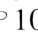

A- Proper Alignment of Mountain Pose (Tadasana)

- Stand erect with chin parallel to floor.
- Draw shoulders back and down away from ears.
- Bring tips of shoulder blades down toward hips and open chest.
- Press feet into ground allowing the knees to face forward.
- Raise kneecaps and engage muscles.
- Lift torso from hipbones to top of shoulders.
- Lengthen tailbone downward toward feet.
- Spread fingers apart and press palms together.

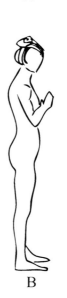

A

B- Improper Alignment of Mountain Pose

- Neck is not aligned with curvature of the spine (extended).
- Shoulders lean forward straining neck muscles.
- Upper back arches, excessively weakening thoracic vertebrae.
- Hipbones lean forward, causing the tailbone to tip backward,
  creating posterior rotation. Posterior rotation causes all joints superior
  and inferior, from the pelvis, to weaken and become susceptible to bone
  deterioration.

B

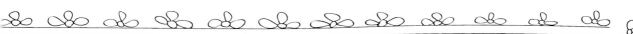

 ## Proper position of the Shoulders and Shoulder Blades

Observe the diagrams below and study the position of the shoulder blades.

Image 1 demonstrates what happens to the shoulder blades when the back muscles begin to weaken. As the muscles supporting the shoulder blades become fatigued. They spread away from the spine and shift in a forward direction. This causes the upper body to appear slouched. The problem is not the neck or shoulder muscles causing misalignment, but the muscles that derive from the back.

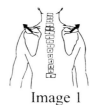

Image 1

To correct this misalignment, the back muscles need to be restored. Trapezius, Erector Spinea and Latissimus Dorsi are the large powerful muscles holding the spine in a healthy alignment. Unfortunately, when these muscles are neglected they become weak and fatigued. Ensure better support and stronger alignment by drawing your shoulder blades together and down.

Image 2: The scapulas are in proper alignment, located toward the middle of the back and toward the center of the spine.

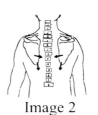

Image 2

Image 3: Proper posture displayed, pull your shoulder blades together and down. Focus your mind on the tip of the blades, marked with an "X." Attune your mind to a single point in this part of your body and learn to contract these muscles. This locks your posture in perfect alignment every time. Good posture is like plugging your body into a circuit. When your spine is properly aligned, the spaces between the vertebrae "open," allowing blood to heal every cell in your body. Good posture helps you feel great!

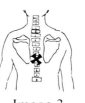

Image 3

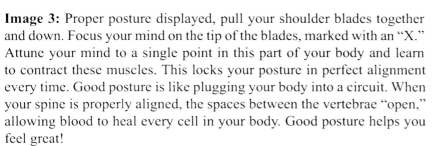

Centering your Balance

Wall Yoga is about centering. Centering your balance is the ability to be continuously aware of the distribution of your weight in relationship of the gravity of earth. Pressing your hands into the wall or binding into a twisting position all involve centering. If you observe the poses that are selected in the book, you'll see they're chosen to help develop the art of centering.

To center your balance, simply close your eyes and begin to acknowledge the relationship between the weight of your body and the gravity of the earth. Begin to develop a sensation of the pressure in your feet against the floor. Learn to shift the weight within your feet evenly from the back of the heel to the corner of your small toe. Then extend medially to the opposite corner of your big toe. This is the beginning of centering your balance.

First you align your body, then you center. Repeat this cycle until you achieve the best alignment. Once you feel centered, and your pose is stable, you will be able to enjoy the transition between steadying your pose and "letting go". Letting go simply means to lighten your body weight and feel as though you are floating in your asana.

Centering your asana is mentally, spiritually, and physically beneficial. "The Art of Centering" will take you on a journey of bringing you back 'home', connecting your body and mind to the present.

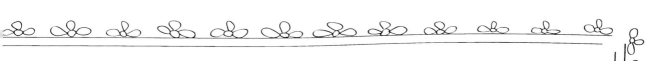

 Engaging your Torso

In the standing position, engaging your torso involves gently contracting your abdominal muscles, rib muscles and stretching your spine. To contract your abdominals muscles, gently recede the navel toward the back of the spine then gently "zip up" the lower abdominal muscles as though slipping on a pair of well-fitted jeans. Engaging the ribs is to draw the sides of the rib cage toward the center of the spine and gently pull downward. Imagine someone wrapping their arms around your torso and giving you a gentle hug.

Learn to feel the muscles under your arms contract. This will help maintain a healthy engagement from your hips to your shoulders. Once your torso is engaged, begin to envision an imaginary string lifting your entire torso from the base of your tailbone to the top of your head.

Maintain this alignment while keeping your chin parallel to the floor and tailbone slightly tipped inward.

As you apply this stature, you'll begin to feel an amazing sense of energy and poise in your body. By elevating your spine, you are physically creating "space" between each vertebra where the blood can freely flow to and from the spinal cord providing life and energy to all your cells. Transportation of blood to all the organs and tissues in your body is the most powerful antidote you can have to heal and live well.

Locate the Focal Point

The focal point is found where you center your body weight in your asana. This place is usually a joint, the connecting cables of the entire body. Whether it's the joints of the neck, shoulders, hips, hands, or feet; when our joints are weak our whole body is affected. When you practice your asana, begin to position your body so you can place as much weight as you can comfortably sustain on the focal point.

For example, when applying the Extended Legs Binding Series, once your body is aligned, begin to draw your body weight to the hip of the folded leg you are resting on.

Tendons and ligaments within the joints are very strong and tough. They are designed to support your frame. Unfortunately, when they get tight they can be very stubborn and immobile. By effectively stretching this area, you release tension and heal the surrounding tissue. Flexible joints play a crucial role in the health of our body. When our joints are healthy, our entire body is able to move with ease.

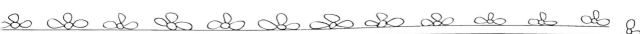

 Flexibility of the feet

There are 26 bones and over 100 ligaments in the foot. This makes up a very complex and perfectly balanced mechanism. They flex forward, back, and side–to–side, supporting your entire weight. Needless to say, the design and science of how the feet work in relationship with the ever-changing body weight they bear, is nothing less than a miracle. This is why it's critically important to keep our feet functioning and healthy down to the smallest toe.

Yoga is a wonderful way to care for our feet and help them maintain flexibility and movement. From my own 30 years of experience in bodywork, if your feet are happy, your entire body is happy. When practicing yoga, stay attuned to the placement of your feet. Avoid straining your ankles or toes when setting your balance. Healthy feet depend on a well-balanced body and the body likewise depends on healthy feet.

When using the downward dog or similar poses where the toes are flexed, take advantage of this opportunity to exercise and strengthen the intricate muscles of the feet that support the joints and bones in each toe. Toes keep our body balanced and our movement fluid. When flexing your toes in your asana spread your toes evenly apart, down to the last toe, then press the balls of your feet into the earth. See the diagram below. By flexing your feet in this powerful exercise, you will keep your toes and arches strong and supple. This prevents stiffness and arthritis that occur when joints are immobile.

The picture to the right is a sample of pressing the balls of your feet into the ground in a Crescent Lunge (Alan asana) Pose. As you sink deeper into the lunge, occasionally allow your body weight to shift to your back foot. Concentrate on spreading your toes into the floor, which will help strengthen these delicate bones and stretch tight muscles and ligaments.

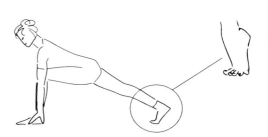

Energizing your Body

Staying focused over a period of time can sometimes be challenging in your yoga workout. Periodically, you need to "energize" your hands or feet. Allowing the energy within you to extend to the very tips of your fingers and toes will help you focus. In yoga, always stay in a state of focus and guard your mind and body from becoming sluggish in your asana. It's certain when your fingers and toes are energized your entire body will function at its optimum level.

 ## Creating a Flow

As you become familiar with each asana and understand proper body alignment, you will begin to move from one asana to the next without having to interrupt the flow. In Sanskrit, the meaning of flowing from one movement to the next with synchronized breathing is called Vanyasa.

To help enhance this flow, mentally visualize the process step-by-step so your body and mind can maintain the rhythm. As you become familiar with each pose, you can incorporate your own workout to keep your body and mind challenged. Be sure to alternate forward poses with back bend poses so you can experience a total body workout. Pay special attention to the pattern of your breathing and ensure each inhalation and exhalation becomes your guide as you flow from one asana to the next.

Colette's Sacred 7 Principles of Enhancing your Yoga Experience

In my studio, I have developed these 7 sacred principles to promote healing your body and calming your soul. Each principle is detailed in the following pages.

1. Breathing

2. Power of Grounding

3. Favorable Attitude

4. Youthful Spine

5. Power of Muscle Memory

6. Engagement

7. Asana Lockdown

1. Breathing

"And God breathed into his/her nostrils the breath of life, and Thus became a Living being."
— **Genesis 2:7**

Do not underestimate the power of breathing. Extend every breath to its full capacity. This is the most natural yet promising tool to enhance your yoga experience. There is no other form of exercise that values and respects the power of breathing through yoga. The Bible says "God breathes breath into man and woman." Breathing is the force that brings death to life. In yoga, this force is celebrated.

Breath is a gift. When practicing yoga use your breathing as a tool to help concentrate. As you breathe life into your body, imagine your breath as living energy washing and transforming your mind and body. Anything alive is in constant motion. As you breathe your body is changing. A new breath means new energy is entering your body. Learn to keep your muscles relaxed and passive while breathing. Let your entire body be energized.

One popular breathing technique you can use during your yoga practice is called "Uijayi Breath". Uijayi Breath means "victorious" breath. It has the ability to build physical endurance. This method consists of narrowing the air passages in your throat. By constricting this muscle called the epiglottis, it enables you to control the flow of air on inhalation and exhalation. Concentrate on the sensation and duration of your breath. This enables your mind to maintain focus and calm your body.

Use your Uijayi Breath as a guideline in flowing from one asana to the next. Soon you'll experience a powerful life force energy called *prana*. Learning proper alignment takes time, as does developing full and steady breathing. On inhalation, allow your breath to permeate into a deep steady flow from your chest to your lungs to your abdomen. Feel the pressure of your breath against your ribs pressing forward, back and sideway without raising your shoulders. On exhalation, slowly release the air, gently guiding your breath steadily and evenly.

As your asana transforms, your breathing pattern will alternate. Never assume you've mastered the skill of breathing. You'll lose the opportunity to grow and learn. Breathing is a spiritual teacher. Listen and learn.

2. Power of Grounding
"Focus: It is a process of diverting one's scattered forces into one powerful channel."
— James Allen

Grounding trains your mind to focus and your body to become centered. To mentally ground, you must use all your senses to experience the full quality of grounding your asana. When you apply your mind and body to yoga, amazing things happen. Grounding your pose gives you the ability to manage your mental and physical well-being. It pulls you from feeling scattered and overwhelmed, to being focused and in control.

When you feel secure in your foundation, you can stretch further and reach farther. One powerful way to reinforce grounding is using the sense of touch. Touch is very effective in allowing you to maintain a focused mind. When you position your body in your yoga practice, acknowledge the surface that your body is in contact with. Whether it's the Wall, Floor, Therapy Ball, Yoga Knots or Yoga Blocks, let your body, hands and feet feel the texture and stability of its surface.

Grounding your asana allows your muscles to relax. When this occurs it opens the opportunity in your asana to stretch more deeply reaching tight muscles and ligaments within the joints. When you penetrate to this level, your body alignment transforms into a higher state of overall well being.

When grounding, acknowledge the magnitude of the earth and trust your body to surrender its support. When you do, you can let go of fear and anxiety. Grounding surrenders you to a place of incredible strength.

3. Favorable Attitude
"Yoga is the perfect opportunity to be curious about who you are."
— Jason Crandell

A favorable attitude means taking life into a "divine" realm. It is living with enthusiasm. You create a vision for positive self-awareness, and what you desire in life. You achieve total acceptance of who you are. A favorable attitude gives you the strength to be true to yourself. You live life with the passions of your convictions from your inner compass. Favorable attitude is the state of thinking the extraordinary, and living the exceptional by erasing negativism and doubt.

The Impossible, gives way to The Incredible.

We all have a "calling" in our lives. It begins by permitting our mind to explore our vision of possibility, and embrace what we believe is destined for us. One of my favorite examples is Jesus. He lived above the ordinary circumstances of his daily life, never wavering in his vision of what he knew was his "calling."

Yoga is a wonderful vehicle in helping us to experience this liberating state of mind. Your mind and body learn to tune into the powerhouse of where your inner potential resides. At my studio, I instruct my students to make a conscious effort to deliberately "step into" a higher place when they "step onto" the mat. As you do, you release all negative thought and emotion that oppress and debilitate you. Use your yoga session as a place to learn and grow physically, as well as, spiritually. All of life's finest ingredients are available to you when you inherit a favorable attitude.

4. Youthful Spine

"Yoga is the fountain of youth. You're only as young as your spine is flexible."
— **Bob Harper**

One way youth is measured is by the flexibility of the spine. As bodies age, the spine becomes less mobile. Practicing yoga is a powerful remedy for treating a stiff, tight spine. Your spine is made up of three natural curves: the cervical (neck), thoracic (mid back), and the lumbar lordotic curve (low back). These segments act like a shock absorber keeping your spine loose and supple.

Think of the spine as a tall brick building. Once the building deviates from the center every brick above and below the structure is affected, causing the entire building to suffer. When this happens the spine's natural curve begins to compensate causing the vertebrae, muscles and the disks between the vertebrae, to weaken. Eventually, the spine becomes stiff and immobile, making it susceptible to degenerative conditions such as arthritis and osteoporosis.

To prevent such havoc, our spine needs to maintain its proper alignment. It needs to have the ability to rotate in its full range of motion. A healthy spine is capable of bending 90 degrees forward, 30 degrees backward and 30 degrees laterally (sideways). By the time we're 40, many have lost more than half this range.

Applying the 'Art of Centering' found in Wall Yoga can help regain this mobility. The asana I have selected for this book involve twisting and revolving; not only to maintain flexibility but to lift and separate each vertebra. When we "open" the spaces between our vertebrae (called intervertebral spaces), we allow the blood to flow more efficiently which is healing every tissue in the body.

Thoracic Issues

One section of our spine that can become excessively tight is the middle upper back, or thoracic. The thoracic is sometimes known as the fulcrum of the spine. A fulcrum is a point or support on which a lever pivots. Much of the spine's mobility depends on the flexibility of the thoracic region. Often emotional and physical stress will go directly to this vulnerable area causing tightness and stiffness.

Other factors that hinder the mobility of the thoracic spine are gravity and locked shoulder blades. Over the years, constant pull and stress in this area causes the curve to continue to exaggerate backwards. This can eventually lead to a stooped posture often referred to as "Dowagers Hump." Shoulder blades help to protect the thoracic spine, but unfortunately they are also a major factor in hindering thoracic mobility. When the muscles under the blades such as the *Sub Scapularis* and *Rhomboids* become tight it is very difficult to loosen these muscles.

Stiff shoulders and neck contribute to immobility of the thoracic region. To break through this barrier, deep and powerful yoga poses that involve flexing, extending and rotations are crucial to restore the flexibility of the thoracic area of the spine. Periodically, in my yoga classes, the majority of our session will involve loosening up the mid back between the shoulder blades. Working through this barrier eventually allows nourishment and mobility to heal all the vertebrae and intravetrebral spaces along the spine. As the spine heals, muscles, joints and all the organs within your body begin to be restored.

A flexible spine creates more movement to your shoulders, elbows, fingers, hips, knees, feet and toes. Be an advocate for your spine and consciously stretch to full capacity when practicing your asana.

5. The Power of Muscle Memory
"We are fearfully and wonderfully made."
— Psalm 139:14

Muscle memory is the body's amazing ability to "remember" a repetitive muscular movement. We rely on muscle memory everyday of our lives. How to walk, swim or brush our teeth is all granted to us by the unique chemical mechanism of muscle memory. Muscle memory involves the mind interpreting an image, processing the image, then allowing you to perform the image.

How can we apply this to improve and advance our yoga workout? When attempting a new asana or perfecting a previous one, you must use your mind in combination with your muscles. Correct alignment means having your feet planted and in line with knees, knees in line with hips, hips in line with shoulder, etc.

First, your mind must recall a properly aligned asana. With muscle memory, you want your mind to imprint only an accurate pose. Eventually, as muscle memory is established and your muscles become stronger, you'll be able to hold your pose for five or more breaths. Lastly, muscle memory requires "faith."

Although your muscles may not be cooperating, your mind is still working.

By the end of 30 days, if you've been following the Wall Yoga program faithfully, your asana will be steadier and solid. You'll feel an amazing change in your body and mind.

Muscle memory is a powerful tool. Trust this process and let it work.

6. Engagement

"When meditation is mastered, the mind is unwavering like the flame of a lamp in a windless place."
— **Bhagavad-Gita Gita**

Engagement is the final step in applying a solid asana. When you engage your muscles, you are simply applying an isometric contraction. Isometric contraction is a form of exercise, which involves the static contraction of a muscle without any visible movement in the joint. This form of exercise is extremely powerful and effective in elongating and strengthening muscles. Isometric contractions are also very effective in cleansing the muscles of toxic buildups and waste.

You attain your asana so you can engage your muscles. Engagement moves you beyond simply holding your pose ---*to embracing it*. To engage your muscles, first position your asana in proper alignment. Then gently contract the muscles that are involved in sustaining the asana such as your legs, or arms or torso. Engaging also includes applying root locks or Bandha. Bandhas produce a particular effect on your physical energy. They increase physical strength, develop muscular control and support your spine.

We mention two types of Bandhas here. They are the Mula Bandha and Uddiyana Bandha. Mula Bandha consists of lifting the pelvic floor muscles. The result is a feeling of core strength in the body, and a mental/physical lightness. Uddiyana Bandha, or upward flying lock, refers to lifting your low abdominal muscles (beneath your navel).

To apply Uddiyana Bandha, gently draw the muscles beneath your navel inward and upward replicating a scooping effect. Bundha are especially effective in conjunction with the Uijayi Breath to create an internal heat within your body. This internal heat is known to have a strong cleansing and purifying effect on your body. It burns away mental, emotional, physical and spiritual debris.

Applying isometric muscle contraction helps build and tone muscle tissue without fatiguing or damaging muscle fiber. The application of engagement with the root lock creates an effective tool to center and balance the body. By applying engagement or isometric contraction, muscles are contracted in their natural state, which reinforce proper joint alignment. When joints are properly aligned, bones and ligaments move in a pain free, fluid motion, restoring health, vitality, and muscle tone.

7. Asana Lockdown
"Yoga is difficult for the one whose mind is not subdued."
— Bhagavad-Gita

When you are setting up your poses, there is a sequence you should follow to ensure a powerful, effective asana. This is why it's important to develop a mental checklist to observe during your early stages of practicing yoga.

Remember, your checklist will vary slightly from pose to pose but the objective remains the same. Your list should look something like this:

1. Lock abdominal core, navel inward and upward (Bandhas)
2. Draw shoulder blades toward center and downward
3. Engage and energize muscles in arms and legs
4. Gaze, gently toward focal point
5. Breathe steady and focused
6. Balance your center
7. Liberate and let go

Repeatedly review your checklist while reestablishing, repositioning, and redefining your pose. Learn to always approach all your asana with strength and vigor and you will reap the reward.

Conclusion

When you prepare for a yoga workout, indulge yourself in a place of quiet and calm. Yoga is a promising oasis to mend your body and strengthen your soul.

Review my Sacred 7 Principles. They are invaluable tools to help you progress in your yoga. There are a lot of things in this world that are uncertain but when you include yoga in your life, you create an environment of consistency and stability. Just as a child needs consistency to feel loved, you need consistency to feel centered, internally and externally.

With yoga, your life becomes better. You have more respect for yourself and thus love yourself more. In yoga, nothing is forced; it's about reclaiming the essence of who you are, what you feel, and where you are in your life's journey. I tell all my students, "Love yoga, and love yourself." With self-acceptance, the desire to eat well and care for your body comes naturally. Loving yourself unconditionally cultivates miracles within you and people around you.

Yoga is about taking control of your life and living it passionately. Gradually, the caring for your body and eating healthy becomes a joy and an honor. This is not hype, just fact.

Life, like breath, is a gift. Learn to take it in fully.

Wall Yoga
The Art of Centering

5 Week Progress Chart

Week 1   _____

Week 2   _____

Week 3   _____

Week 4   _____

Week 5   _____

USE THIS PAGE TO CHART YOUR WEEKLY PROGRESS

Cut & Display

Week One

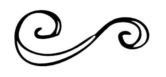

Day 1   Flat Back Pose   _____

Day 2   Chandra Pose   _____

Day 3   Boat on Ball Pose   _____

Day 4   Downward Dog Leg Kick Pose   _____

Day 1

Flat Back Pose

1
- Bend Forward at Hips, Hands on Wall
- Open Legs, Bend Knees
- Press Chest Toward Floor

2
- Place Left Hand on Block
- Lift Tailbone to Ceiling
- Engage Arms & Torso

Advanced

Cat & Cow Stretch

Cow
- Kneel on All Four
- Lift Head and Tailbone Toward Ceiling
- Lower Abdomen to Floor

Cat
- Raise Spine to Ceiling
- Tuck in Tailbone and Bring Chin to Chest

31

Chandra Pose

1

- Kneel, Chest Open, Blades Down
- Hands in Prayer Position
- Press Thumbs to Heart

2

- Place Left Foot on Floor, Right Toes on Wall
- Open Arms Wide, Shoulder Height
- Engage Torso

Advanced

Extended Arm Stretch with Yoga Knots

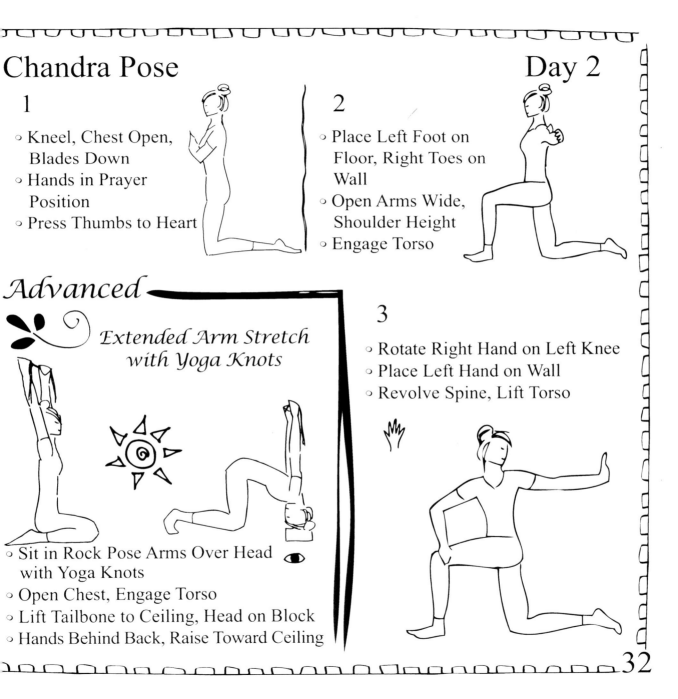

- Sit in Rock Pose Arms Over Head with Yoga Knots
- Open Chest, Engage Torso
- Lift Tailbone to Ceiling, Head on Block
- Hands Behind Back, Raise Toward Ceiling

3

- Rotate Right Hand on Left Knee
- Place Left Hand on Wall
- Revolve Spine, Lift Torso

32

Day 3

1

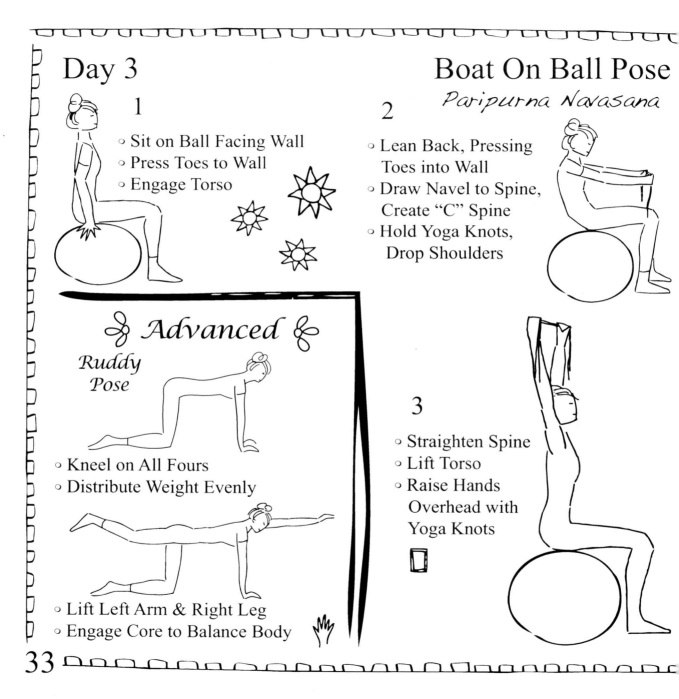

- Sit on Ball Facing Wall
- Press Toes to Wall
- Engage Torso

Boat On Ball Pose
Paripurna Navasana

2

- Lean Back, Pressing Toes into Wall
- Draw Navel to Spine, Create "C" Spine
- Hold Yoga Knots, Drop Shoulders

Advanced

Ruddy Pose

- Kneel on All Fours
- Distribute Weight Evenly

- Lift Left Arm & Right Leg
- Engage Core to Balance Body

3

- Straighten Spine
- Lift Torso
- Raise Hands Overhead with Yoga Knots

Downward Dog Leg Kick Pose

Adho Mukha Svanasana

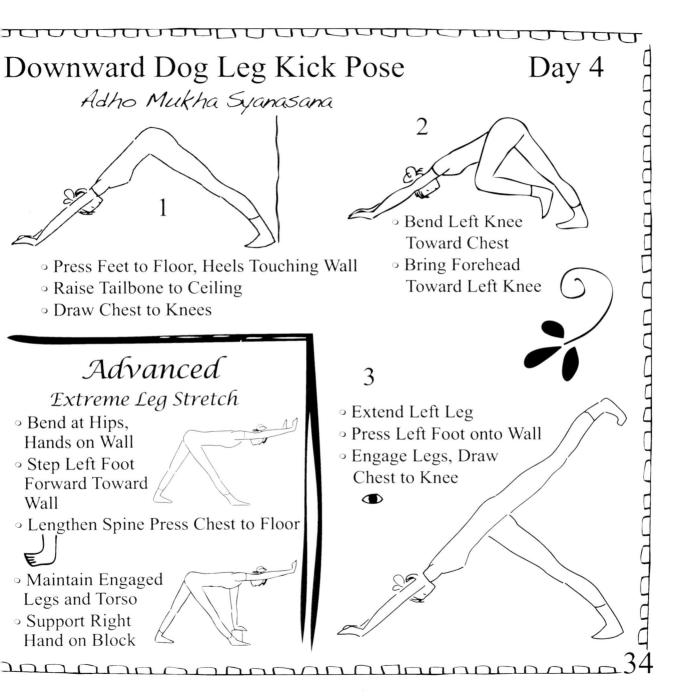

1
- Press Feet to Floor, Heels Touching Wall
- Raise Tailbone to Ceiling
- Draw Chest to Knees

2
- Bend Left Knee Toward Chest
- Bring Forehead Toward Left Knee

Advanced
Extreme Leg Stretch
- Bend at Hips, Hands on Wall
- Step Left Foot Forward Toward Wall
- Lengthen Spine Press Chest to Floor

- Maintain Engaged Legs and Torso
- Support Right Hand on Block

3
- Extend Left Leg
- Press Left Foot onto Wall
- Engage Legs, Draw Chest to Knee

Week Two

Day 1

1

- Sit in Rock Pose, Face Wall
- Blades Rolled Back, Chest Open
- Chin Leveled

2

Balsana

- Lean Against Wall, Raise Elbows to Wall
- Lean Chest Forward, Rest Hands on Shoulders
- Pull Blades Together and Downward

Advanced

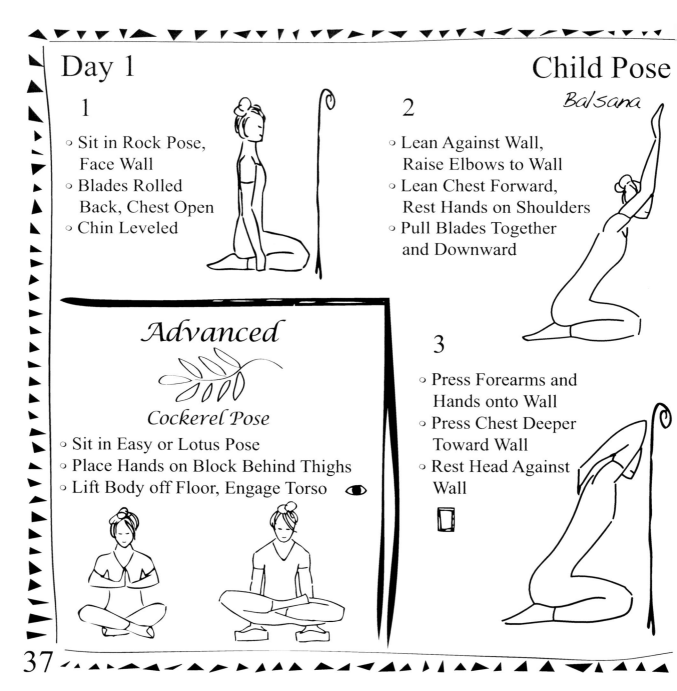

Cockerel Pose

- Sit in Easy or Lotus Pose
- Place Hands on Block Behind Thighs
- Lift Body off Floor, Engage Torso 👁

3

- Press Forearms and Hands onto Wall
- Press Chest Deeper Toward Wall
- Rest Head Against Wall

Extended Side Angle On Knees Pose

Utthita Parsvakonasana

1
- Sit on Floor
- Right Hand Next to Wall, Legs Rest Under Left Arm

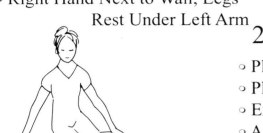

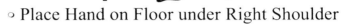

2
- Place Hand on Floor under Right Shoulder
- Place Left Hand Behind Back
- Extend Left Leg Laterally from Body
- Align Left Shoulder to Left Hip to Left Foot

Advanced
Half-Bound Lotus

- Sit on Floor, Fold Left Foot on Top of Right Thigh
- Pull Left Foot in with Yoga Knots
- Extend Right Hand, Touch Toes
- Fold Chest Toward Knees

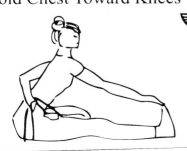

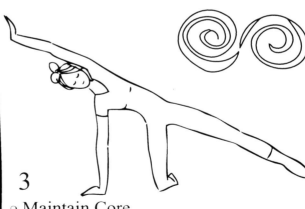

3
- Maintain Core
- Extend Left Hand to Wall, Away from Left Foot
- Stack up Shoulders to Shoulders and Hips to Hips

38

Day 3

Forward Bend With Ball Pose
Uttanasana

1
- Lay Backwards on Ball
- Arms Extended Overhead
- Chest Open, Feet Press Wall

2
- Lift Body with Abdominals
- Fold Body Forward
- Wrap Arms, Press Feet on Wall

Advanced
Leg Toner on Ball
- Press Hands into Corner of Wall
- Lift Legs High to Ceiling
- Engage Legs and Buttocks

3
- Continue to Engage Abdominals
- Fold Body Toward Knees
- Press Feet to Wall

Dancer's Pose
Natarajasana

1
- Mountain Pose, Hands Pressed Together
- Raised Torso, Chest Open
- Feet Pressed to Ground

2
- Maintain Engagement
- Lift Left Leg, Balance Body
- Left Hand Holds Left Foot

Advanced
Crocodile to Baby Cobra
- From All Four, Lower Body
- Chin, Chest, Knees and Toes Touch Floor

- Unfold to Baby Cobra
- Shoulders Back, Head Raised

3
- Press Right Hand on Wall
- Continue Raising Torso
- Left Hand to Inside Left Foot and Raise to Ceiling
- Lift Torso Upward

40

Week Three

Day 1

Utkatasana

1

- ○ Bend Knees, Toes under Feet
- ○ Chest Open, Blades Down
- ○ Tailbone Toward Floor

2

- ○ Engage Torso
- ○ Hands in Prayer
- ○ Tailbone to Floor, Eyes Forward

Advanced

- ○ Maintain Core
- ○ Arms Raised over Head
- ○ Chest Open, Blades Back

3

- ○ Press Hands onto Wall
- ○ Maintain Core
- ○ Feet Press to Ground

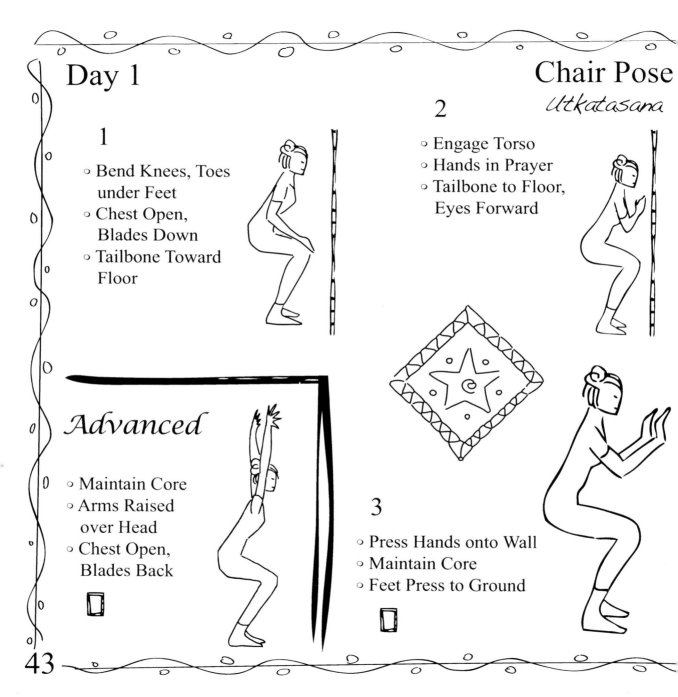

Spinal Twist Pose

Ardha Matsyendrasana

1

- Squat on Toes in Prayer Pose
- Keep Chest Open, Right Shoulder Facing Wall
- Engage Torso

2

- Twist Body Toward Right, Palms on Wall
- Engage Torso
- Press Left Hand into Wall, Twist Deep

Advanced *Extended Leg Binding Series*

- Sit with Right Knee Folded to Chest, Left Leg Extended

- Extend Right Hand, Lean Chest Forward

- Wrap Right Hand Outside, Right Leg, Left Hand Grabs Yoga Knots

Day 3

1

- Rest Body Forward on Ball
- Press Feet into Floor & Wall

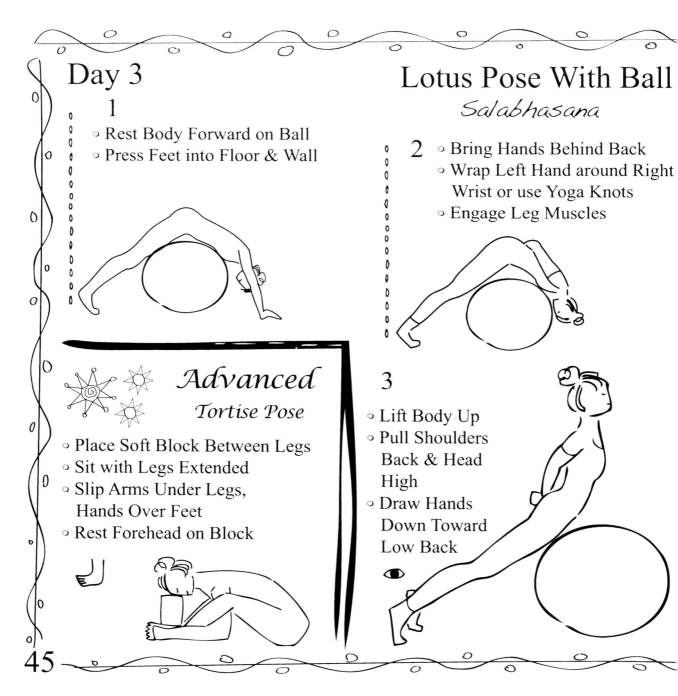

Lotus Pose With Ball

Salabhasana

2

- Bring Hands Behind Back
- Wrap Left Hand around Right Wrist or use Yoga Knots
- Engage Leg Muscles

Advanced

Tortise Pose

- Place Soft Block Between Legs
- Sit with Legs Extended
- Slip Arms Under Legs, Hands Over Feet
- Rest Forehead on Block

3

- Lift Body Up
- Pull Shoulders Back & Head High
- Draw Hands Down Toward Low Back

Extended Side Angle Pose
Utthia Parsvakonasana

1

- Stand in Mountain Pose, Press Hands to Chest
- Chest Open, Draw Blades Downward
- Engage Torso

2

- Facing Wall, Place Hands on Hips
- Step Left Foot Toward Wall
- Balance in Deep Lunge

3

- Place Left Elbow on Left Knee
- Reach Right Hand over Head
- Press Right Hand into Wall
- Reach Right Hand Reach Toward Ceiling

Advanced
Revolving Leg Stretch

- Fold Right Leg Against Body
- Extend Left Leg
- Place Block Outside Left Knee
- Left Elbow on Block, Reach Toward Ceiling

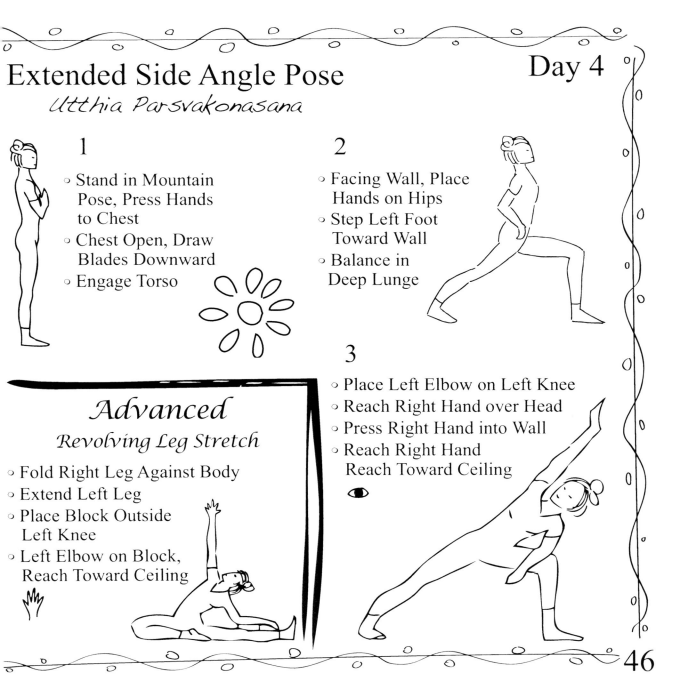

Week Four

Day 1

Half Moon Pose
Ardha Chandrasana

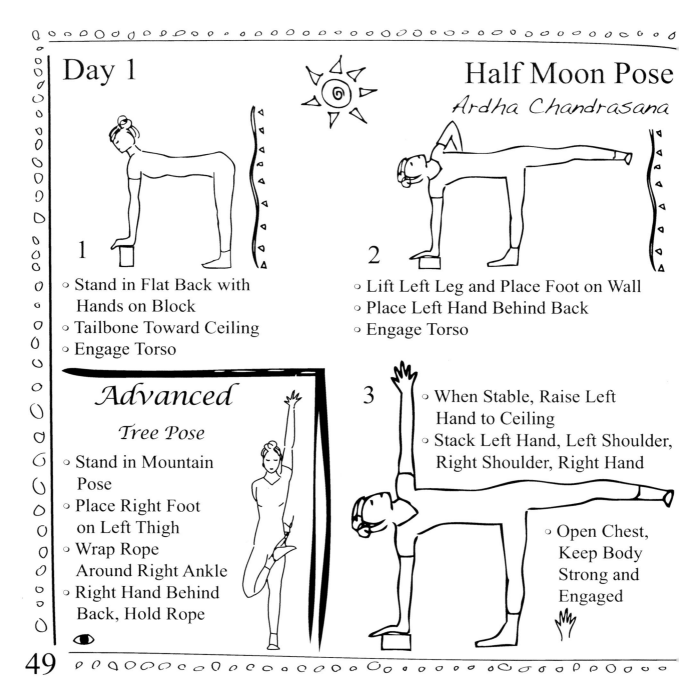

1
- Stand in Flat Back with Hands on Block
- Tailbone Toward Ceiling
- Engage Torso

2
- Lift Left Leg and Place Foot on Wall
- Place Left Hand Behind Back
- Engage Torso

Advanced
Tree Pose
- Stand in Mountain Pose
- Place Right Foot on Left Thigh
- Wrap Rope Around Right Ankle
- Right Hand Behind Back, Hold Rope

3
- When Stable, Raise Left Hand to Ceiling
- Stack Left Hand, Left Shoulder, Right Shoulder, Right Hand
- Open Chest, Keep Body Strong and Engaged

Triangle Pose
Utthita Trikonasana

Day 2

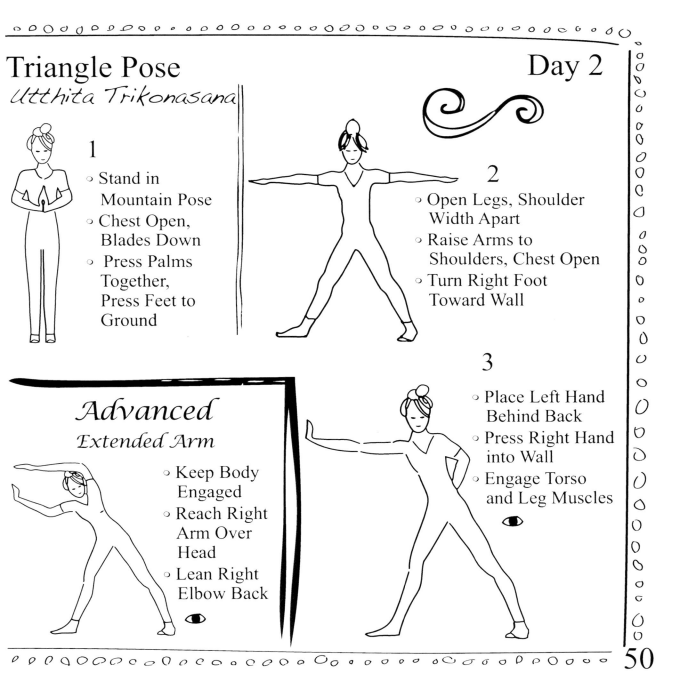

1
- Stand in Mountain Pose
- Chest Open, Blades Down
- Press Palms Together, Press Feet to Ground

2
- Open Legs, Shoulder Width Apart
- Raise Arms to Shoulders, Chest Open
- Turn Right Foot Toward Wall

3
- Place Left Hand Behind Back
- Press Right Hand into Wall
- Engage Torso and Leg Muscles

Advanced
Extended Arm
- Keep Body Engaged
- Reach Right Arm Over Head
- Lean Right Elbow Back

50

Day 3

Lateral Incline Pose On Ball
Vasisthasana

1
- Press Right Hip on Ball
- Right Hand Behind Head
- Press Feet into Wall

2
- Extend Left Arm Toward Wall
- Press Feet into Ground
- Engage

Advanced   *Seated Forward Bend*

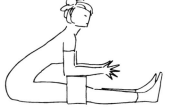

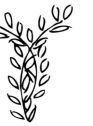

- Sit With Legs Extended
- Lean Forward at Hips
- Elbows on Blocks, Gaze Forward

- Sit With Legs Extended & Open
- Lean Forward at Hips
- Elbows on Blocks, Gaze Forward

Shoulder Stand Pose

Sarvangasana
"Queen of all Asanas"

1
- Lay on Yoga Blanket
- Lift Legs Over Head
- Lift Torso Toward Ceiling, Place Hands on Back
- Press Feet onto Wall

2
- Steady Body, Engage Torso
- Raise Right Foot to Ceiling
- Steady Left Foot on Wall

Advanced
Eastward Pose

- Lie on Floor, Rest Sacrum on Block
- Place Right Foot on Floor, Left Foot on Wall
- Rest Body
- Lift Both Feet on Wall ◉

3
- Raise Both Legs to Ceiling
- Engage Legs and Torso, Point Toes
- Support Torso with Hands ◉

Week Five

Day 1	Modified Beam Pose	_____
Day 2	Monkey Pose	_____
Day 3	Plank on Ball Pose	_____
Day 4	Upward Facing Bow Pose	_____

Day 1

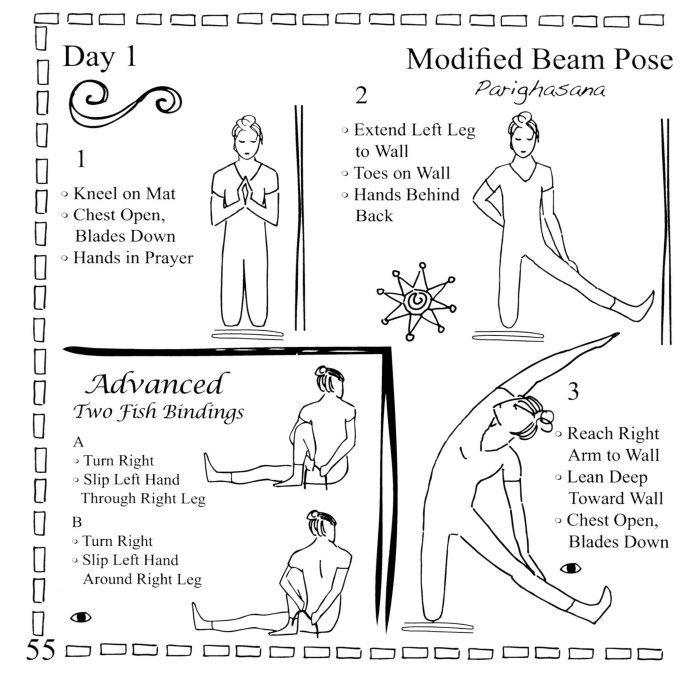

1

- Kneel on Mat
- Chest Open, Blades Down
- Hands in Prayer

Modified Beam Pose
Parighasana

2

- Extend Left Leg to Wall
- Toes on Wall
- Hands Behind Back

3

- Reach Right Arm to Wall
- Lean Deep Toward Wall
- Chest Open, Blades Down

Advanced
Two Fish Bindings

A
- Turn Right
- Slip Left Hand Through Right Leg

B
- Turn Right
- Slip Left Hand Around Right Leg

Monkey Pose
Hanumanasana

1
- Stand in Flat Back
- Legs Bent ot Straight
- Chin Lifted, Blades Down

2
- Fold into Forward Bend
- Chest Toward Knees
- Crown of Head to Earth

3
- Raise Right Leg up onto Wall
- Press Toes onto Wall
- Fold Body Close to Wall
- Keep Both Legs Strong

Advanced
Tiptoe Pose

- Stand, Right Ankle Across Left Thigh
- Bend Right Knee, Hands in Prayer

- Bend Forward
- Lean into Right Leg
- Hands on Floor or Blocks 👁

Day 3

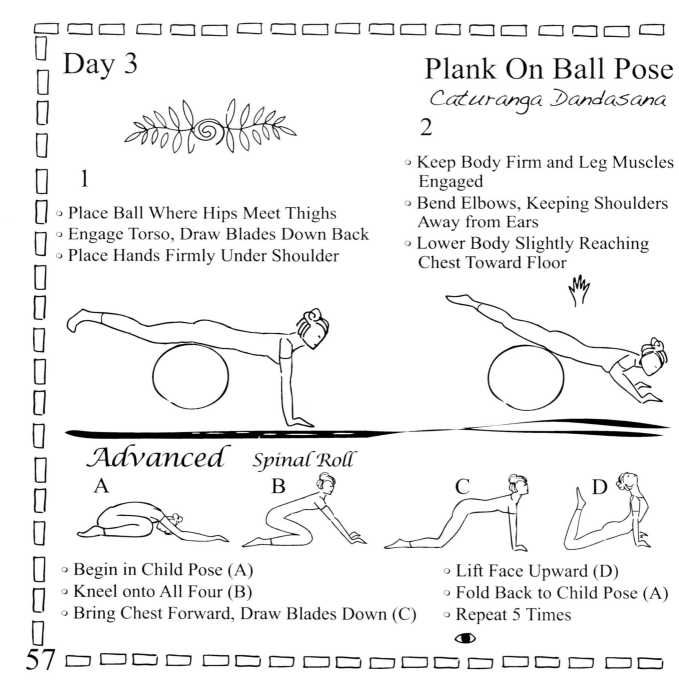

Plank On Ball Pose
Caturanga Dandasana

1

- Place Ball Where Hips Meet Thighs
- Engage Torso, Draw Blades Down Back
- Place Hands Firmly Under Shoulder

2

- Keep Body Firm and Leg Muscles Engaged
- Bend Elbows, Keeping Shoulders Away from Ears
- Lower Body Slightly Reaching Chest Toward Floor

Advanced *Spinal Roll*

A   B   C   D

- Begin in Child Pose (A)
- Kneel onto All Four (B)
- Bring Chest Forward, Draw Blades Down (C)
- Lift Face Upward (D)
- Fold Back to Child Pose (A)
- Repeat 5 Times

Upward Facing Bow Pose

Urdva Dhanurasana

1
- Place Block Next to Shoulders
- Lie on Back
- Feet on Floor, Arms Next to Hips

2
- Place Hands on Block Next to Shoulders
- Push Torso Toward Ceiling
- Place Top of Head on Floor

3
- Raise Torso Up to Ceiling, Arms Extended
- Engage Shoulders and Legs
- Tip Head Back

Advanced
Cow Face
Gomukasana

- Cross Left Leg on Top of Right Leg
- Pull Feet to Sides
- Push up with Blocks or Raise Arms with Yoga Knots

58

The Importance of Nutrition - *A Message From Philip Barry, D.C.*

Nutrition has always been important to me as any of my patients, colleagues, family and friends will tell you. In this feature, I am going to give you simple steps to take charge of your health and vitality. As a chiropractor, I primarily focus on function rather than symptoms. Patients frequently come to me looking for the proverbial "magic bullet" or the latest fad.

There is no magic bullet. Health and wellness are more than the latest exercise, vitamin remedy or diet. The patients I treat who have the most success at recovering or reinvigorating their lives tend to do five things better than my patients who don't follow the guidelines I've outlined below.

My favorite example is a hand. It has five fingers. A hand with less than five fingers is incomplete and thus cannot function normally. My 30 years of experience and training in the Chiropractic approach to medicine has revealed that we as human beings cannot function normally without five facets of health and wellness in balance. They are:

1) Good Posture
2) Proper Nutrition
3) Adequate Rest
4) Proper Exercise
5) A Positive Attitude

When these five facets are implemented properly, health and vitality return and improve. The trick is to know how to implement these concepts. My insight is not the "sexy" answer people want to hear. Nor is it filled with flamboyant and exaggerated claims where one can lose fifty pounds the first week, or look and feel fifty years younger after one workout. But my program works. The concepts are proven and have stood the test of time. So let's get started. Stick with me. You'll be glad you did.

Yoga, in my professional opinion, is the best way to train the muscular support system of the body. Why is good posture important? Good posture reduces stress on the spine including the muscles and importantly the nervous system. People with good posture in their day to day activities sustain less injury, miss less time from work and generally feel better on a day to day basis. This is due to the decreased stress on their nervous system, especially the nerves exiting the spinal column. If you faithfully do the program outlined in this book your posture will improve. Mine did.

Good posture is not automatic. It is not the result of being strong or having the strongest muscles. Good posture has more to do with "training" the muscles that support us as opposed to strengthening the muscles that hold our body upright. It has everything to do with muscle memory. Strong muscles in many cases are tight, inflexible muscles. Heck, I've been to the gym and I've seen some of the strongest guys brandishing the worst postures. I know you've seen it too.

My second area for change is nutrition. We have all heard you are what you eat. What we take into our body forms the building blocks of our entire body, and how it functions. The food we eat affects us all the way down to our molecular cell level. Here's my next point. Write it down and don't forget it.

THE FOUNDATION OF EVERYONE'S DIET SHOULD BE PLANT BASED.

What does this mean? It means when you eat a meal your decision needs to be "What shall I eat with my salad?" Plants need to be the foundation of every meal. This is a fundamental, but necessary, shift in thinking. Here's why: coronary artery disease is the leading cause of death in both men and women in the United States. In the U.S., more than a half million people die of it every year.

The pace of the American life style drives the food industry in the United States to mass produce and deliver tasty, high processed, fat laden foods on demand. In order to overcome this lifestyle, we must be willing to make a paradigm shift in diet. A plant–based diet works by providing micronutrients. These are found in the highest concentration in green leafy vegetables.

Vegetables provide a plentiful source of enzymes and trace minerals. Vegetables contain phyto chemicals. These are natural chemicals beneficial to human health. Vegetables also contain complex carbohydrates, fiber, protein and healthful fats such as omega 3 fatty acids, which aid digestion.

In my practice, many of my patients lament about mistakes they've made with food choices. I encourage them to focus on good choices. For more information on how micronutrient deficiency results in disease, and ways to eat for optimum health, feel free to check out my blog at www.wallyogaworkout.com

The third factor is your body needs down time, quality down time. Our body heals itself when we are sleeping. Not sleeping well can cause disease. The most common problem my fibromyalgia patients complain about is the inability to get enough sleep. Lack of sleep can lead to diseases like depression and lack of focus at work. Did you know that physical activity that occurs while exercising leaves the muscles relaxed whereas prolonged mental activity leaves the muscles tense? In other words, proper exercise such as yoga helps us to sleep better.

When you don't sleep well, you don't get enough rest and fatigue results. Your performance at work suffers, and interpersonal relationships decline, creating stress. Yoga decreases stress and helps us to sleep better, reversing the trend. I have found certain herbs, minerals and vitamins aid in gaining proper sleep. Did you know that valerian root extract is known for calming nerves and promoting restful sleep without unpleasant side effects? Did you also know that a magnesium deficiency can cause leg cramps at night and that magnesium can actually produce a calming effect on the brain allowing for a more restful sleep?

Fourth, I think that we all realize that we need exercise. Many times though I treat patients who have started an exercise program and they FEEL WORSE! What's up with that? Well, exercise must increase strength and flexibility at the same time, which is where many exercise programs fail. Indulge me for this quick example: we all hear terms like "the strong armed quarterback" or "the baseball pitcher who can throw one hundred miles per hour." Are these guys huge and muscle bound? No, many times they are long and lean like Tom Brady of the Patriots, or Randy Johnson of the Diamondbacks.

Likewise, we need to build long lean muscles that are flexible and allow our joints full range of motion. Joints that move freely remain healthy longer. I'm a proponent of functional training. I don't favor working out muscles individually because I don't believe that it leads to proper biomechanics and function. I see more people out of balance as a result of exercising muscles individually than not. The exercise training that I have seen get the best results are Yoga and Pilates.

Finally, we've heard all the adages about a positive outlook on life. The bottom line is no one gets well unless they want to! I see it in patients all the time. Some patients make remarkable recoveries. They respond faster and better than I ever imagined. Why is that? They want health and vitality! They aren't going to let anything stop them. They follow my advice, and don't miss a day of exercise. When they start feeling better and getting stronger, it motivates them to achieve more success.

One easy way to be successful is a simple self-affirmation of your values, goals and aspirations by reciting daily affirmations. It's easy to get off track. Don't let the distractions around you thwart you from your goal. The spirit is willing but the flesh is weak. I see it all the time with people trying to lose weight. Well, there is help and this book may be the first step. Yoga not only improves your body balance and physique, it gives you the ability to sleep better and be more rested. It can even have an effect on your brain chemistry (endorphin production) which can alleviate symptoms of depression and fatigue, decrease reliance on medications to regulate your mood.

I recommend yoga to all my patients and I see miraculous results every day. There you have it my friend.

Yoga, it's powerful, plug in.

Dr. Philip Barry, D.C.   drphilip@wallyogoworkout.com

61

Wall Yoga
Charts and Routines

Before you begin this next chapter, you must understand proper alignment using proper breathing techniques. In this chapter, yoga routines are introduced to help you begin to understand and apply various poses in conjunction with breath. Forward bends, back bends, revolving poses and balancing poses are all components that help you experience a total workout with grace and ease.

As one asana flows into another, your mind and body become quiet and focused, reserving the necessary energy to heal and mend your body. As in the Sun Salutation and " Wall Yoga" routine, you can repeat this exercise as often as you wish. Learn to enjoy the repetition, which will allow your body to stress less on perfection and surrender more into rhythm and flow.

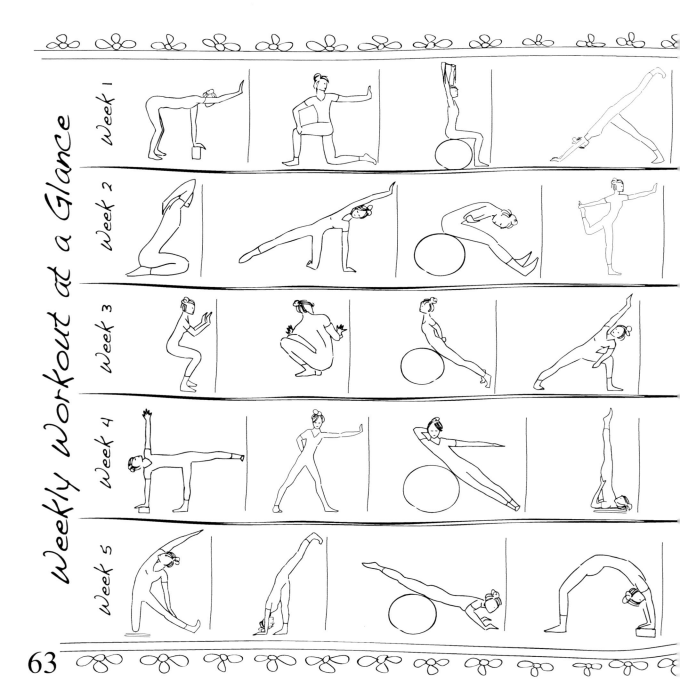

Weekly Workout at a Glance

Week 1
Week 2
Week 3
Week 4
Week 5

Wall Yoga Routine

This routine gives you the opportunity to practice moving from one pose to the next using a steady breathing pattern. It helps build change to concentration and edurance, creating flexibility for the spine. Follow the sequence first with the right leg and arm, then repeat with the left leg and arm.

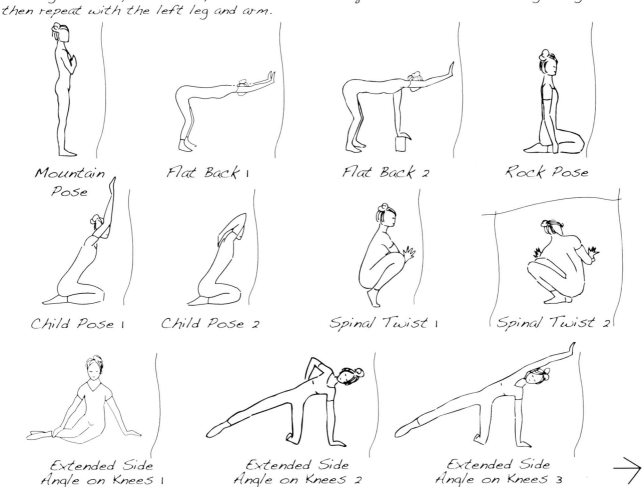

Mountain Pose

Flat Back 1

Flat Back 2

Rock Pose

Child Pose 1

Child Pose 2

Spinal Twist 1

Spinal Twist 2

Extended Side Angle on Knees 1

Extended Side Angle on Knees 2

Extended Side Angle on Knees 3

→

Wall Yoga Routine
(continued)

Extended Arm
Stretch 1

Extended Arm
Stretch 2

Cat Pose

Cow Pose

Downward Dog
Leg Kick 1

Downward Dog
Leg Kick 2

Downward Dog
Leg Kick 3

Mountain Pose

Dancer's Pose
Against the Wall 1

Dancer's Pose
Against the Wall 2

Mountain Pose

Spine and Hip Opener Routine

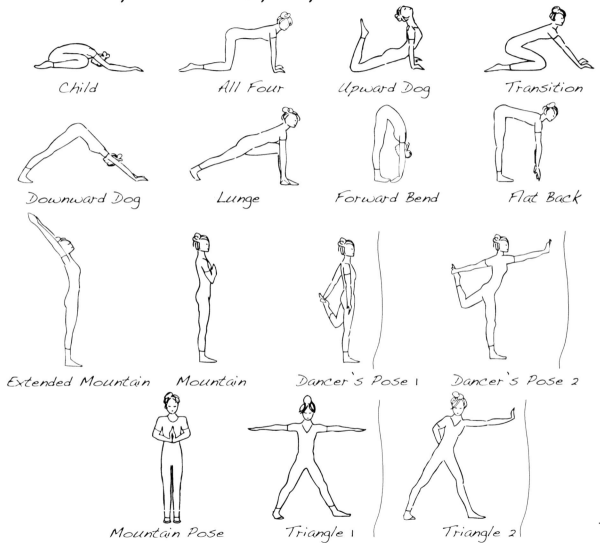

Child

All Four

Upward Dog

Transition

Downward Dog

Lunge

Forward Bend

Flat Back

Extended Mountain

Mountain

Dancer's Pose 1

Dancer's Pose 2

Mountain Pose

Triangle 1

Triangle 2

→

Spine and Hip Opener Routine
(continued)

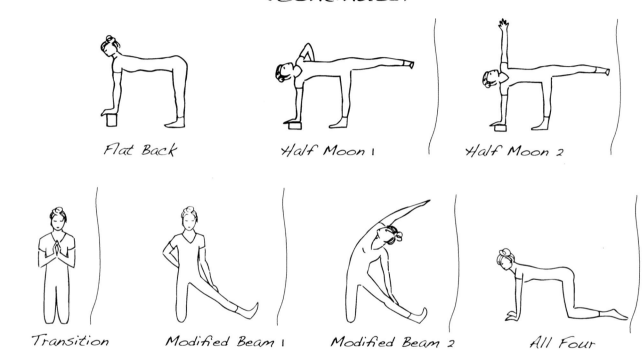

Flat Back

Half Moon 1

Half Moon 2

Transition

Modified Beam 1

Modified Beam 2

All Four

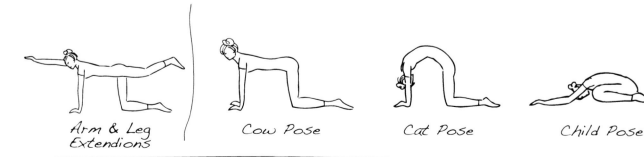

Arm & Leg
Extendions

Cow Pose

Cat Pose

Child Pose

Wall Yoga on Ball Routine

Ball exercise is an excellent workout that quickly helps build your core and balance. This complete workout includes Forward Bends, Back Bends, Lateral Bends and relaxation. Concentrate and flow from one pose to the next. Practice each pose 5 times and increase to 10 reps on each series. Synchronize your breathing to the flow. Follow the sequence first with the right leg and arm, then repeat with the left leg and arm.

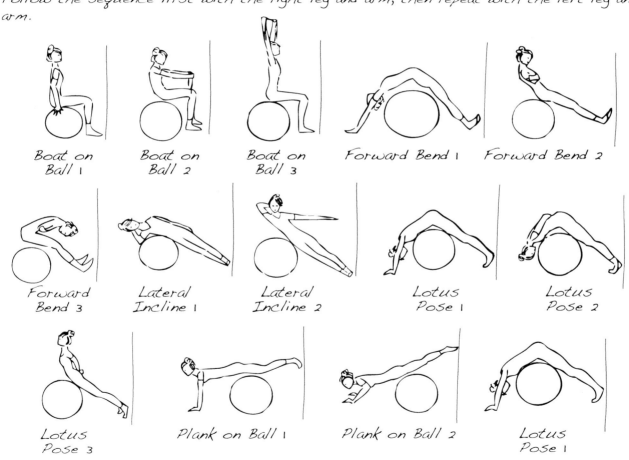

Boat on Ball 1

Boat on Ball 2

Boat on Ball 3

Forward Bend 1

Forward Bend 2

Forward Bend 3

Lateral Incline 1

Lateral Incline 2

Lotus Pose 1

Lotus Pose 2

Lotus Pose 3

Plank on Ball 1

Plank on Ball 2

Lotus Pose 1

Sun Salutation

This modified Sun Salutation is a beautiful sequence that can be used as a warm-up or cool-down. This series is so powerful it can also be used on its own. Follow the sequence first with the right leg and arm, then repeat with the left leg and arm. Synchronize your breathing to the flow.

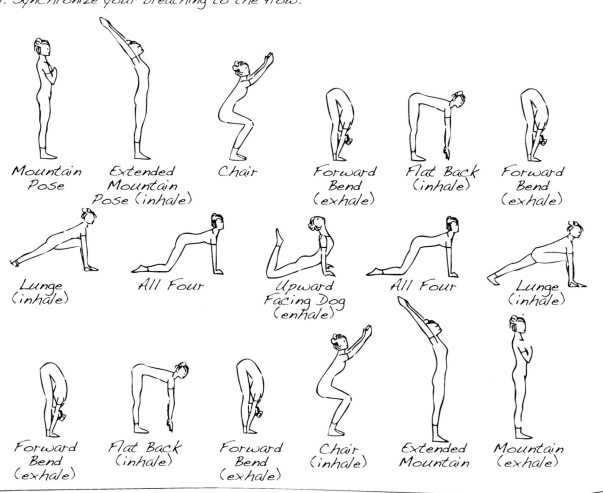

Mountain Pose

Extended Mountain Pose (inhale)

Chair

Forward Bend (exhale)

Flat Back (inhale)

Forward Bend (exhale)

Lunge (inhale)

All Four

Upward Facing Dog (enhale)

All Four

Lunge (inhale)

Forward Bend (exhale)

Flat Back (inhale)

Forward Bend (exhale)

Chair (inhale)

Extended Mountain

Mountain (exhale)

Suggested Readings

Thai Yoga Massage by Kam Thye Chow, Healing Arts Press, Vermont 2004 - "Thai Yoga Massage is practiced as a duet. Counterbalancing and levering the recipient's body with his own, the practitioner works with gravity, breath, and directed touch to create a harmonious and therapeutic "dance" with the recipient. This imparts physical vibrancy, grace, and spiritual energy" Wonderfully illustrated and easy to follow, it can be applied on one another during Yoga practice.

Total Astanga by Tara Fraser, Duncan Baird Publishers, London 2005 - This book is beautifully illustrated and offers many modifications to help achieve a fulfilling yoga practice. Frasers takes you step-by-step through each posture in the primary series. Wonderful for beginners as well as advanced students.

Chakras Energy Plan by Anna Selby, Duncan Baird, UK 2006 - A must have for all beginners in studying Chakras Energy. It will help you regulate your energy flow with safe, effective techniques and routines. Includes yoga and chi gong postures, meditations and visualization. It's very encompassing.

Yoga Mind and Body by Sivananda Yoga, Vedanta Center, Dorling Kindersley Limited, London 1998 - The holistic approach to health, vigor and happiness, through the five disciplines of Yoga - proper exercise, yogic breathing, proper relaxation, vegetarian diet and meditation.

Hatha Yoga Illustrated by Martin Kirk, Brooke Boon, Daniel DiTuro, Human Kinetics, IL 2006 - Experience the physical benefits and body awareness from hatha yoga, the most popular form of yoga today. Hatha Yoga Illustrated presents nearly 650 full-color photos to visually demonstrate 77 standard poses from hatha yoga. These apply to all major hatha styles including Iyengar, Astanga, Anusara, and Bikram.

Visit our online store to purchase any of these items- www.WallYogaWorkout.com

Music

Paint the Sky with Stars by Enya- Enya's voice is so enchanting and soothing. It's perfect to lift your soul while participating in your yoga session or meditating. Enya reaches into your soul and makes you feel wonderful. It's much more than a musical experience! There are 16 songs and all of them are great. It's perfect for the best of yoga album. I find it great for stress relief. I could not recommend it more highly.

Memory of Trees by Enya- Enya's voice is very mesmerizing and beautiful. She seems to be a one-woman band accentuating a very moving, inspiring melody. It's wonderful to play while practicing yoga. The music has the ability to calm and energizes your mind and body at the same time. A must for all Celtic lovers.

Scottish Moores/Emerald Isle by Lifescapes- Some of the best Celtic music I've ever heard! It's never tiring. This music is inspiring, breathtaking, sensual and uplifting. It's wonderful to play during Yoga a perfect compliment. This music is simply brilliant.

Sacred Earth Drums by David and Steve Gordon- My favorite for percussion. Its magical and very healing. The nature sounds with rain sticks, flutes and drums is just fabulous! The songs have rich melodic beats. A real joy to listen to. The drumming is being used these days in therapies as a tool of reconnection and wellness (see the book, "The Healing Power of the Drum" by Robert Lawrence Friedman). This CD takes us to that connection. Its great and highly recommended! It's terrific for an energizing Astanga workout.

While participating in your yoga session or meditating, Enya reaches in your soul and makes you feel wonderful.

Visit our online store to purchase any of these items- www.WallYogaWorkout.com

Products

Soft Yoga Blocks by Nu Source- Excellent yoga blocks that offers solid support but still have some "give." Rare to find, soft Yoga blocks you can comfortably rest your head or spine on. We have various Yoga blocks in our studio yet "Soft Yoga Blocks" are everyone's "favorite."

Thera Ball by Nu Source 65cm- A 55 centimeter round inflatable ball used for stretching and developing flexibility for better physical fitness. Included is an easy to use hand pump so you can take your exercise balls with you wherever you go. This ball will enhance your workout giving you results. Ideal for stretching, strengthening and toning exercises.

Yoga Mats by Europa- 5mm & 6mm Thick Yoga Mat- Europa Mat is made in Germany by one of the world's leading manufacturers. This textured mat has a dry grip which is great for wide angle poses. The Europa Mat is certified under Oeko-Tex Standard 100 product class IV, which meets human-ecological requirements to be safer for all skin contact. It is also fungal and bacteria resistant. Available only in size 24" X 68." Great to cushion knees and head.

1/4" Extra Thick Deluxe High Density Yoga Mat by Yoga Accessories- At 6.2mm, our extra thick yoga mat is a full 1/4" thick, and is one of the thickest mats on the market. The mats come in a variety of colors that are strong and vivacious, but not overpowering in their brightness. This well-made yoga mat will add comfort to your yoga workouts. And because of its high quality, this mat will last longer than most standard foam mats. When shopping around for a yoga mat, note that what many other companies call a 1/4" mat is actually 4.5 - 5.2 mm in thickness -- considerably thinner than this mat.

Yoga Knots from "Wall Yoga"- Natural cottoned weaved ropes 1/2" in diameter intermittently arranged with knots to assure a more solid grip. Colorful hand painted woodens balls are attached at both ends.

Yoga Gloves and Socks by Yoga Paws- Mini yoga mats for your hands and feet! These small mitts fit right over your hands and the balls of your feet and make it possible to practice on just about any surface! Yoga Paws are made from a unique non-slip material (nylon/polyvinyl blend) that is similar to the material of a yoga mat, but with perforated holes to allow your skin to breathe. Adjustable Velcro closure ensures a proper fit. Includes a complimentary carrying bag. Excellent for travel and a great idea for home practice on carpet or the wall! One order of Yoga Paws includes 4 pieces: 2 for the hands and 2 for the feet. Available in regular size (for most women), and large size (for most men).

Visit our online store to purchase any of these items- www.WallYogaWorkout.com

Testimonials

When I was diagnosed with Limb-Girdle Muscular Dystrophy, I felt that my time being ambulatory was like sand through an hour glass. As the years passed, my body began failing me and I would fall unexpectedly and often. I assumed it must mean that my time outside of a wheelchair was creeping up behind me. Then, I was introduced to yoga. Initially, I laughed at the idea. I thought to myself, "That's something reserved for celebrities and otherwise healthy, strong individuals!" I never thought I would have been able to do it, but I was very wrong. These simple, controlled movements have done wonders for me. I'm no longer out of touch with my body. My coordination has improved. I fall a lot less. Living with a disease for which there are no treatments and no cure, this is more than I could have ever asked for. I tried both physical and occupational therapy for some time, and never got these kinds of results.

In addition to feeling more physically stable yoga has been an unexpected gift. Stretching and opening up areas of tightness such as my hips, back and shoulders improved my physical and mental well-being. I immediately feel better after a yoga session. It is not unreasonable to say yoga has become my drug of choice. I plan on doing it as long as I am able, and in my heart, I know that doing these simple things for myself will buy me years of mobility. It has also helped me to appreciate what my body can do, rather than yearn for what it cannot. I can't describe the mental peace that brings. If you have any kind of physical disability, I strongly urge you to try Colette's system. I never thought I would be able to do any exercise regime outside of a hospital setting, and here I am, 2 years later, feeling better and stronger. I am forever grateful for finding this. My life is better because of it.
- Kelsey G.

Miracle Worker
"You are a miracle worker! I can not, nor can I ever put into words beyond this...You have saved my life. And now I let others know what you are doing for me. And that if they too wish to survive they must at all costs, pursue these same endeavors. It did not take me long to realize that it does not take you long to realize what your students need. Even when we the students don't know."
- Pat H.

Getting Back My Life
"I'm so glad you have been a blessing to me. You are so patient and positive. You clearly explain what you want me to do. You encourage me. You set reachable goals. You tailor the work to fit me, you give me personal attention to the minute detail. You make me feel successful when I might otherwise be upset with the weakened condition of my body these days. You always reward my effort which makes me want to try harder. You explain why the techniques are important. You explain the benefits to my body of what we're doing. your facility is beautiful. On and on and on, Thank You! Thank You! Thank you!"
- Troy M.

Author Biography

Author and Illustrator, Colette Barry is a licensed Massage Therapist of 30 yrs. She is also a certified Yoga Instructor at Yoga Alliance, a certified Pilate's Instructor and Thai Yoga Therapist.

Growing up, her father practiced Chiropractic Medicine. Here Colette came to understand the art of holistic healing through her father's passion for his patients. From an early age, she began working with her father treating a multitude of ailments, from chronic low back pain to Multiple Sclerosis and Muscular Dystrophy. Having terrific success in her massage practice, Colette took her unique theory of body mechanics and incorporated it into her Yoga and Pilates practices.

The combined result was nothing short of amazing!!

Colette has been recognized many times over the years in countless forums via TV/radio, newspaper/magazine articles and now the web.

"Wall Yoga, The Art of Centering", is Colette's first book. Her hand-rendered art brings warmth to every page as you turn through the cleverly sketched poses (asana) detailed there. She offers you an inviting 'peek inside' to come and experience Yoga...on your own terms.

Today Colette and her husband, Dr. Philip Barry D.C., C.C.S.P., own and operate a thriving Health Clinic, in the heart of Westlake, OH. It is here that they "branded" their own unique form of training and conditioning with the best of today's Yoga and Pilate's programs.

In addition to her work in her studio, Colette is a mother of three beautiful children, a devoted spouse and a friend to many. Her Yoga and Pilates programs continue to blossom with new students delighted to add Colette's unique programs to their regular weekly workouts. Her step–by–step instructions from her new book, "Wall Yoga, The Art of Centering", are a must see!

Visit Colette online and experience the genuine warmth that will buoy you through your day.

Live happy. Be well ... Namaste

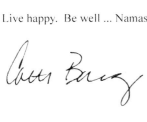

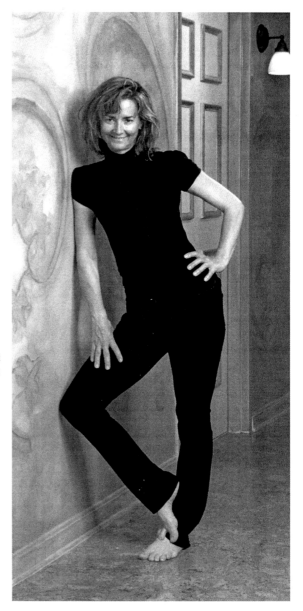